HOW MY MOM'S
STAGE 3B CANCER
WAS CURED

Joanna Narum

INTRODUCTION

My mom was diagnosed with stage 3B lung cancer in November of 2002. It is now 2014 and she has been CURED of cancer since February of 2004. I am writing this guide in hopes that people who have cancer or a family member with cancer will see what was done to cure my mom's cancer and hopefully be able to employ the same techniques to cure themselves or their family member. My mom's cancer was said to be incurable and also the most difficult type of cancer to survive when she was first diagnosed, so I want this book to serve as real hope for cancer patients that it is possible that they too can beat cancer and become healthy again. Cancer does not have to be a death sentence. It can, and has been beaten by many, many people.

I have written the exact methods we used to facilitate my mom's cure in the first half of the book so that you and your family can begin to use the same techniques as soon as possible. Then, the rest of the book will chronicle the weekly emails my dad had sent to friends and family updating them on my mom's progress and the ups and downs we endured during her illness. I have also included some of the helpful and supportive responses we received during this time and the words of advice and encouragement which we found helpful as well.

I certainly hope that this guide will help you and your loved ones through the very difficult time you are enduring, and that the techniques we used on my mom will also be used by you and that you are successfully and permanently cured of cancer! My mom has been cured for 10 years now...and she is living proof it can be done. My best wishes to you and your family, and may you have total success in your cure.

Chapter 1

"No evidence of malignancy". This was the report we got back from the doctor on February 13, 2004, after a year and 3 months of worry, anguish, fear and ups and downs. My mom had been diagnosed with stage 3B lung cancer in November of 2002. It is now January of 2014, and I am delighted to say my mom has been cancer free for 10 years! I wanted to write down exactly what was done to make my mom's cure possible, in hopes that this book will help many more people be cured of cancer also.

When my mom was diagnosed, the doctors said it was not curable. They said she likely wouldn't survive a year and that her chances of survival were 15% that she'd live for 5 years. Thanks to my dad's refusal to accept those statistics, we got to work and thank God my mom was cured. I have wanted to write this book ever since, because I hope to help other people with cancer and their families and hope that they too, will be cured.

My mom had been in good health all her life until 2002, when her voice became hoarse and it wouldn't go away. At first, we thought it was a cold, or just a sore throat, but when it didn't get better, she went to the doctor and they took x-rays, did a CT scan and finally a scope, which is an instrument with a camera on the end that the doctor uses to see inside the patient. The scope revealed a suspicious lump under her bronchial tube. It was pressing on her vocal nerve which was therefore causing her hoarse voice and difficulty talking. The doctor then took a biopsy of her lung, and it came back as cancerous....not operable....too close to the aorta and windpipe to risk operating on. The doctor said her only options were to have chemotherapy and radiation, although soon after these initial appointments the doctors my mom was seeing disagreed as to whether she could survive having it surgically removed or not. The doctors said mom's cancer would be very hard to remove surgically because it involved the lymph nodes in the middle of her chest which are very hard to get. Mom had smoked since she was a teenager, but ironically had quit just a year before this. Now, the doctors were saying she had cancer. STAGE 3B LUNG CANCER. Stage 4 is the worst, and lung cancer is known to be the toughest of the cancers to cure. We were terrified for her.

After my parents received the diagnosis, they called a family meeting where they told the rest of us what they found out. My dad has always been a very organized person, so he had taken notes at my mom's appointments thus far and had all the information there with him as he told us the horrible news. I remember it as though it were yesterday, all of us in our parent's living room, my mom on the couch, my dad in his favorite chair (he had a brown easy chair he always sat in to read the paper, etc.) and the rest of us in various spots around the room. He said: "you know mom's been having a hoarse voice in recent weeks, so we went to the doctor to have it checked out and...........it's CANCER." My heart dropped to my feet as he said it. Even with no details yet, everyone knows that cancer, any kind of cancer, is very bad news. My dad proceeded to give us the details that it was stage 3B lung cancer, it's inoperable and that she would have to undergo chemo & radiation starting right away. Our family all hugged my mom and said we will beat this. My dad had not yet told us all the grim statistics on survival that he had been informed of at the doctor's office, but when we found out about them we chose from the beginning to IGNORE those statistics and decided to do whatever we could to overcome this and beat the cancer.

As I looked online that night, I saw article after article that said "lung cancer is the hardest cancer to beat and anything stage 3 or higher is virtually impossible." I kept searching, though, hoping that some article SOMEWHERE on there would say stage 3B lung cancer IS curable, but I never did find it. I kept searching and searching, thinking that if at least one article said it, I could have real hope that she will be cured. But there was no such article. I then decided that although we have an uphill battle to endure, and although the statistics were against us, we needed to do everything we could to cure mom. And this is what we proceeded to do.

CHAPTER 2

For the last couple of years, I've worked at a health products store in a call center where we take calls from customers who are ordering vitamins. I get to talk to many wonderful people from all over the U.S., and some share their stories of having a friend or family member with cancer. Each time I got one of these calls, I shared the story of my mom's cure and the ingredients that made it possible. They were always relieved and had renewed hope after I told them the doctor's grim diagnosis in the beginning, their depressing prediction of her future and their astonishment when the cancer was gone!

One older man called who had stage 4 lung cancer. He said he has the will to fight but the doctors kept saying it's very unlikely he can survive. I wish doctors wouldn't do this to patients, because many people take the doctor's word as final and always right and they are NOT always right. They should not diminish or destroy people's hopes by saying discouraging things. People need to believe they can get well and ignore any grim statistics and predictions they come across. Doctors are wonderful in many ways, but this hopelessness some of them cause by telling patients these depressing predictions of doom are not at all helpful. If we had listened to their prognosis for my mom, we would've gone home and essentially waited for her to die. Instead, we decided to do whatever it took to cure her. By the time I told the man who had stage 4 cancer the story of my mom and how she was cured, he had renewed hope and told me "you just saved my life". I was so happy to have been able to help him get renewed hope and vitality to fight and destroy the cancer!!

It was then I knew I needed to write this book and share the story with as many people as possible. I remember how hopeless we felt when my mom was first diagnosed and how everything we read online and heard from the doctors was discouraging, so I am hoping this book will be the beacon of light you need to know you can survive too! I hope and pray that our ways will help you or your friend or family be cured of cancer forever. So now, to the techniques we used...................

CHAPTER 3

Our first and most important ingredient for my mom's cure was PRAYER. Everyone in my family prayed daily for her to be cured. We told all our relatives and friends about her diagnosis and asked them to pray also. Some of our relatives are very religious, and they put my mom on their churches prayer list too, which we were very thankful for. My dad sent weekly email updates to our friends and relatives so they could know what was going on with her and it also kept her in their thoughts and prayers. All our friends and relatives were so supportive and kind. It was a great help to us.

I cannot emphasize enough the importance of praying for the cancer patient. If your family has not been religious in the past, it is never too late, and you can pray now for God's help. He is ever-forgiving and will accept and listen to all people if they ask for help, even if they have not believed in the past, or feel they are somehow unworthy, or have committed too many sins for God to accept them. He will listen...just pray for his help to cure the cancer. The prayers you say don't have to follow any special protocol, you can simply ask God to hear and help you. According to Pastor Joel Osteen, people often feel they have to speak to God in a special language or using special words and they aren't sure how to go about it, but he says to just speak in your normal way, (politely of course), and thank God for your blessings and ask for the things you need. It doesn't have to be complicated or long winded. Just make it a daily routine and it can work wonders! Daily prayer by you, the patient, and any or all the friends or relatives who will also be willing to pray is crucial.

Now, after the most important part of praying, our next ingredient for my mom's cure was to follow the doctor's recommendation and give her chemotherapy and radiation treatments. The doctors also wanted to surgically attempt to remove the cancer from her lung. They could not agree on the survivability of this though. The cancer on her lung was in a very risky position and could have killed her if there were any missteps. So, at this point, my parents decided to go to M.D. Anderson in Houston, Texas, which is known as the best cancer hospital in the United States.

The doctors there said it was too risky to try to surgically remove the cancer as well. While my parents were in Houston, they visited with their nephew Tim, who lived there, and together they went to Lakewood Church (Joel Osteen Ministries). Our family had watched Joel on television for years before this, and we all think he and Lakewood church are absolutely wonderful. His sermons are always uplifting, and he always speaks of the things that people struggle with on a daily basis. He has good practical advice on ways of thinking that help people excel in their lives and live happily on a day to day basis. He tells stories from the bible that correlate with the lesson he is teaching, and does it in a very inspiring and interesting way. Joel is on television, but it is hard to see his show, because he is always on very early or very late for some reason. He has several books too, so you may want to read those as well. So my parents and Tim went to see Joel on one of the nights when my parents were in town and of course it was a glorious celebration of God and life and optimism which is what Joel is all about! Joel's mom had been miraculously cured of terminal cancer years before as well, and the doctors at the time had written her off. Joel often speaks of his family's good blessings and his gratefulness to God that his mom was cured. This in itself was helpful to us, knowing that Joel's mom had suffered with cancer that was seemingly incurable and she has survived for many years now! When the sermon was over, people from the audience were asked if they would like to come up to the front and pray with prayer partners from Joel's staff. My parents and Tim went up as did many people and waited for their turn in the line they were in. When it was their turn, the prayer partner (his name was Lucky, but we call him Angel), that they got to pray with asked what they would like to pray for today. They told him about my mom's cancer and he said "I hope you don't expect God to cure you." My parents said "That's what we're hoping." And then he said: *"Because he already has."* So they prayed together, standing in a circle, my mom, dad, nephew Tim, and the angel all holding hands. It was such an important and powerful moment just being in such a holy place and having someone from the church so assuredly tell them that she is cured. It made whatever we would have to go through next in the battle achievable. So, after that inspiring visit to Joel's church, they headed home to take on the cancer with chemo and radiation.

My parents also luckily have a friend who is a surgeon, and when they asked his advice on whether to have surgery to remove the cancer, he said "Absolutely not. Surgery is too risky. We can't get it all because it's too close to the aorta. Surgery would weaken the body, the immune system would be compromised and the cancer would spread." My dad researched every possible angle on how to cure my mom. He checked with multiple sources and always had several opinions before they moved forward. Now that surgery had definitely been ruled out, the chemo and radiation treatments were set up and we were ready to begin.

CHAPTER 4

The chemotherapy and radiation began on January 6, 2003. The chemo was done at regular intervals once/week and radiation was done each day for a month until the sessions were completed. Throughout the duration of these sessions we'd take my mom to the hospital and they would hook her up to the machines and she would have her treatments. The chemo/radiation was difficult after the first few sessions because mom felt sick (nauseous), and was not able to eat much at all during this time. Her weight dropped significantly and her hair became sparse. We were very scared for her to be able to eat and maintain strength. The doctors had no solution that was working for this, so my dad found Megace, which is an appetite stimulant, and we gave mom this to help. We had her eat cereal, Boost shakes, Ensure shakes, sherbet and fruit cups whenever she could. They were tolerable to her when all other foods weren't. We used a medicine organizer to keep all moms' vitamins/medications organized so we could make sure she was taking everything she needed to daily. My mom had anxiety during this time, so the doctor prescribed medications to help her with the anxiety and to help her sleep also. The doctors had said that during the first week or two of chemo/radiation there would probably be no problems, then, in the 3rd and 4th week, she would have a sore throat, then in the 5th & 6th week they'd give her pain medication. She was given prescriptions for a variety of medications to help her sleep, eat and reduce anxiety as needed. We would give her the recommended dose, but some made her too drowsy, so we would cut back on those, etc. We learned to keep exact track of each medication she took daily, and if we noticed a pattern of problems, like being too drowsy or "doped up", we would cut back on the ones that were causing problems. The plastic medicine organizer is crucial for medicine organization, and it's best to have someone fill it every Sunday for the next week. Keep track in a notebook of everything they take on a daily basis and note how they felt that day. My dad learned to read the blood tests, and got used to keeping track of mom's white blood cell count. When they were low, we reinforced them with immune building supplements to keep the immune system strong. The doctors said there would be many people involved to help during mom's treatments. My mom had to go into the doctor's office every so often to have fluid transfusions too, when she got too dehydrated. My mom's last chemo treatment was on February 17th, 2003, and her last radiation treatment was the following Wednesday. After the prescribed amount of treatments had been done, the cancer was effectively shriveled to ash, but that did not mean she was cured. The doctor's view was that the cancer had been destroyed.....temporarily. This by no means meant that she was "cured", but that the cancer could, and most likely would, come back shortly. The doctors were just trying to be honest, and tell us the true situation, not wanting to give us false hope. But it sure was a rollercoaster ride for us. Knowing the cancer was now burnt to an ash inside my mom's lung, but that it also could come back in no time at all, was not comforting. But we continued on and tried our best to keep our positive outlook that she would be cured of cancer forever. All along during the time my mom had cancer, my dad took her to every appointment and always took notes. He asked questions every step of the way and always made sure we were doing everything we could to get rid of the cancer. Here is an email my parents sent our friends and relatives after my mom had completed the first week of chemo/radiation:

Greetings Family & Friends,
Jan 6, 2003

Kathy had her first chemo/radiation treatments today...all went well and Kathy is feeling good. The doctors, nurses, assistants, etc. are all great. They treated Kathy very well. And they explained everything thoroughly. Thank you for all your prayers and support. We appreciate it very much! (written by my dad).

Hi Everybody,

The first day of treatment went so well, I can hardly believe it. I guess I was afraid of it more than I knew. This is a huge relief to me. I know that as time goes on it may not always be this way, but you never know, and getting started has been like a huge cloud lifted for me. All of your prayers and good thoughts have done this for me, and I want to thank you! (written by my mom).

The 3rd important part of our success with my mom's cancer was the natural methods we used. My dad's chiropractor recommended we see a natural doctor, Dr. Wright. Dad took mom to see her right after she was diagnosed with cancer and her treatments were not only necessary for my moms' recovery and cure, but they were very comforting for her as well. Dr. Wright always talked positively about my mom's being able to be cured, and her methods were very relaxing for my mom. This was a great help to us because knowing she was a naturopathic doctor and believed my mom could be cured made all the grim statistics from the conventional medicine world seem to fade away. We knew there WAS hope and another way to do things (the natural way).

Dr. Wright would proceed to help us do the correct things to cure my mom. Whenever we took my mom to appointments at Dr. Wright's, she felt relaxed because she knew the treatments were helpful, and there was no pain or discomfort involved either. Dr. Wright used a machine called a Light Beam Generator on mom which could do a scan over my mom's body and eradicate any cancer cells left in her lung. It was very peaceful and comforting for my mom to have this done. We had also read in a cancer book that it's helpful to have the cancer patient visualize wolves attacking the cancer all the time during their various treatments to help the patient feel strong and motivated as they are being treated. Dr. Wright told us that the destroyed cancer cells were being broken up during her treatments and were then exiting through my mom's lymph system.

Dr. Wright would also tell us to have her take vitamin B complex, vitamin C (1,000 mg and must be mineral ascorbates, not acid), hi-lignan/flax seed fiber, vitamin E, Coq10 (30 mg) in lozenge form if possible, garlic 440 mg, multi-vitamin/mineral tablets, ph powder, stevia instead of sugar, and lots of water. Having no sugar is crucial because it is said to feed cancer. Also, Noni juice and spring water were prescribed as well. You can get all of these things at any natural food store, and/or health products store in your town or online. With the help of Dr. Wright, we felt better and better about my mom's long term success. We had regular weekly appointments with Dr. Wright, and these treatments coincided with the chemo/radiation treatments mom got at the traditional hospital. Mom continued on with Dr. Wright's appointments especially after the traditional doctor's treatments had been finished, and with the help of these treatments, mom was COMPLETELY CURED!!

CHAPTER 5

With the doctor's chemo/radiation, Dr. Wright's naturopathic remedies, and especially God's blessings, my mom was able to be cured of cancer. After the cancer was gone, we went back for check-ups at first once/month, then once she kept passing those tests and showing no cancer, then we went to having check-ups once every 6 months and kept receiving the results "no cancer" to which the doctors were astounded. They fully expected to see the cancer to return after the initial eradication had been completed, and some time had passed. It has now been 10 years since my mom was cured! In fact, we just celebrated her 74th birthday in September, and she is in good health. I have written this guide in the hopes that people who were in our position, suddenly devastated by the news that they, or a family member have cancer, will have hope and faith that they CAN be cured. We were said to be an extremely unlikely case for survival in the beginning, first because it was lung cancer which is the hardest cancer to cure, and then also that it was stage 3B lung cancer, which is a half level better than the worst (stage 4). No matter where you live, you can get and do the same things we did. The chemo/radiation can be done at your local hospital, and the medicine and vitamins we used are available almost everywhere in the U.S., but if you're in a small town, you can get them on the internet too. The praying can be done anywhere and everywhere, and the naturopathic doctor's remedies can be done in many places too. We were extremely fortunate to have Dr. Sharon Wright as our naturopathic doctor, but I'm sure there are many others who are compassionate and knowledgeable in your area too. Natural medicine has become very popular and there are doctors all over the U.S. who can give you the treatments my mom received. In fact, at my job in the vitamin company, many of our customers rely on only natural remedies, not traditional prescription drugs that the doctors give. We took the stance that traditional and nontraditional methods used together was the best route to take for success.

When my mom was diagnosed with cancer and was going through all her treatments we didn't know what to expect of course, and therefore it was very scary. When this happens to a family, all you can think of is how to cure them, and of all the great times you have had together, remembering the fun and happy life you've enjoyed with the person who is ill and how those times could all be over with. My mom has always been very elegant, kindhearted and supportive of her family, so to think that she was possibly no longer going to be with us was devastating. All the Scrabble games, visits to grandma's, fun trips together, delicious meals my mom made at home, going shopping together, and spending time with family was possibly over and it was a very frightening time indeed. But despite our fear, we remained faithful that she could be cured, and in the end, she was. If we had not bothered to do the three steps I've described here in the book, she surely would have died. Instead, she is here with us and we have enjoyed 10 more years with her and we plan to have many more to come! So, no matter how many grim statistics the doctors may tell you, how many depressing articles you read online saying it's "incurable", DON'T LOSE HOPE......IT IS POSSIBLE TO BE CURED and I hope our story on what we did to get rid of my mom's cancer will help you realize that cancer CAN be beaten. NOW GO DO IT!!!!

PART 2

In this section of the book, I will first share some of my favorite quotes from the wonderful Pastor Joel Osteen, then the emails my dad sent to friends and relatives during my mom's illness along with helpful advice and prayers we received during my mom's illness.

My favorite quote is: *"When the going gets tough, the tough get going"* ....and also some I've heard Joel Osteen say, such as:

~~~~*When you make up your mind that no matter what life deals your way, you're going to stay calm and at peace, all the forces of darkness cannot keep you from your success.*

~~~~*If you will trust in God and use your energy to believe instead of worry, then God will turn it around and cause it to work to your advantage.*

~~~~If you will hope to the end, divine favor will come

**The above quotes were taken from Joel Osteen's Daily Inspirations

<u>Exerpts From My Dad's Emails To Friends & Family During Mom's Care....</u>

Jan 6, 2003---Kathy had her first chemo/radiation treatments today....all went well, and Kathy is feeling good. The doctors, nurses, assistants, etc. were all great. They treat Kathy very well and they explain everything thoroughly. Thank you for all your prayers and support. We appreciate it very much. (written by my dad).

Hi everybody, the first day of treatment went so well, I can hardly believe it. I guess I was afraid of it more than I knew. This is a huge relief to me. I know that as time goes on it may not always be this way, but you never know, and getting started has been like a huge cloud lifted for me. All of your prayers and good thoughts have done this for me and I want to thank you! (This was written by my mom).   ---Reprinted from earlier in the book

January 13, 2003---the second week of treatment was pretty hard, but the kids came over and helped us get back on track (food and meds).

January 20, 2003---Today we started Kathy's 3rd week of treatment. We've had some problems because of the aggressiveness of the treatment. We're doing both chemo and radiation at the same time...about as aggressive as it gets. We have added two more medications and two midweek infusions of fluids. Kathy's blood work still looks pretty good, but some numbers are a little low...we're getting shots for that problem and we're watching it closely. The doctors said we're going to check our progress in two weeks and if the tumor has shrunk enough, we'll consider maybe surgically removing what's left of it. On the diet front, we're drinking Ensure shakes, peanut butter and jelly sandwiches along with fruit and vegetables.

My sister came over today for a visit. She survived a bout with Lymphoma last year. She is completely cured, which is about a 1 in 100,000 occurrence. She gave more information on how she survived and we got some good ideas from her. We decided to meet regularly to discuss strategy and drink Noni juice too. We feel more optimistic than ever now. Once again, thank you for all your prayers and support. We really can feel the power off your good wishes.

January 27, 2003---We started our 4th week of treatments today, and all went very well. We took note that Kathy is not losing her hair yet. It usually starts falling out about the 2nd or 3rd week of chemo. We're ready for it if it comes (Kathy has 2 new wigs), but we prefer she keeps her hair! We had some difficulty with our meds this week. We overdosed and Kathy slept Friday and Saturday. With the help of the kids, we adjusted her doses and she is doing just fine. I got angry at our doctor today over the meds, and he said that we are currently in the most difficult part of the treatment and it's a tough time. He also said that the chemo is poisoning the cells, and the radiation is burning the cells in an attempt to kill the cancer. Her voice is getting better, and that could indicate that the tumor is shrinking. Kathy is down to 116 pounds, and she might lose more. We really want to stop the weight loss. We're going to try Megace, it's an appetite enhancer that really works for cancer patients. In closing, it's been a rough week. Thank you for your support...Kathy takes the pain, illness and treatment with a quiet strength that is a wonder to behold. It's a matter-of-fact attitude of "let's get on with it", so we can go on with our normal lives. Meanwhile, I'm running around like a chicken with my head cut off. Good thing I've got her and the kids to straighten me out! That's all for now....

(This next email was sent by my dad to a school friend of my moms' who had emailed expressing support for my mom and also telling us of her own cancer.)........

Dear Friends, Kathy was delighted to hear from you. We were unaware of the bout with cancer that your family has endured. We will pray that you do well in your current treatment regimen. We know the power of prayer and feel it constantly from our friends and family from all parts of the country. Kathy was diagnosed with stage 3B non-small cell lung cancer in November of 2002. We went to the M.D. Cancer Clinic in Houston, Texas, for a 2nd opinion in the hope that they could remove the tumor with surgery. They verified the findings, but said they didn't recommend surgery at this time because of the proximity of vital organs. We returned home for chemo and radiation treatments which started in January 2003. The doctors in Texas said that although they may have a slight technical advantage, if we had surgery there, they felt that the emotional value of being home with our family would be our best course of action. Kathy has her chemo every Monday morning, and she has her radiation every day at noon. Her treatment is very aggressive in an attempt to destroy the tumor and Kathy is a real trooper. She takes the treatment very well and has been very brave and strong throughout. We have a whole new library on cancer, and are becoming very knowledgeable about diet, treatments, nutrition, etc. Thank you for your kind thoughts and prayers. We will turn our entire network of family and friends and their prayers toward you and your current battle. We've had a number of friends who have survived cancer in the past few years. It's amazing how much cancer is out there. Be strong, and our prayers are with you.

Feb 3, 2003---Dear Friends and Family,

Today we started Kathy's 5th week of treatment and encountered our first obstacle. We did a blood test and discovered that her white blood count is low, so we deferred the chemo treatment until next week provided the count is back to normal. The white blood cells count is 2.5, and it should be 4-5. So, we're starting antibiotics to ward off infection. This is one of the side effects of chemotherapy and it's troubling when it occurs. We will keep you posted on Kathy's progress. Thank you for all your support and prayers.

Feb 9, 2003---Visit to Dr. Wright

-Light Beam Generator treatment, plus computer and energy test

-Mom felt MUCH better after treatment

-got more Coq10 in lozenge form/ Mom likes

-we stayed for 3 hours

-Dr. Wright's treatment helped keep Kathy's immune system strong. IMMUNE was the name of the supplement we used to help keep Kathy's immune system strong also

Feb 10, 2003---Dear Friends and Family,

Kathy is down to 110 pounds and holding. That's about what she weighed when I first met her in college in 1959. She's getting tired of the whole routine, but she is heartened by the knowledge that she has to tolerate only one more chemo and seven more radiation treatments. The doctor is planning to do a procedure on or about Feb 24th to check our progress. We need you all to re-double your efforts in the area of prayer and positive thoughts between now and then. The doctors say the tumor could be anything from unchanged to gone. We are praying for the latter. Yesterday, Kathy and I went to see our doctor of natural medicine. Kathy was feeling very tired all day, but, after the treatments she was feeling much better. Kathy's white blood count was still around 2.0 today, but they decided to go ahead with her chemo and continue with the antibiotics. I monitored the blood counts and recommended the next course of action. She will also get a shot to boost her w.b.c. tomorrow, after her radiation. Once again, thank you for all your prayers and good wishes. We are going to give it all we've got in our final week and a half of treatments, and we're confident that we are going to beat this thing.

Feb 17, 2003---

Kathy finished her chemo today and we are elated! Her weight is not only holding as we reported last week, but she's gaining...up to 112 from 110 pounds!

We're trying everything to regain Kathy's health, because you never know what's going to work. I do want to give you all a special thanks for all your prayers and good wishes. I know it's working, because Kathy is responding like never before. She is eating better, she's looking better, and she is better able to take part in healing programs in addition to the standard chemo and radiation. We still have two more radiation treatments….one tomorrow, and one Wednesday, and then we're done. The next step will be to do a cat scan and see how well we did with all this sound and fury. Please keep praying for all those you know who are in need. PS----this is a prayer wheel that was sent to us from a friend. Kathy found it very comforting and meaningful…..

Father, I ask You to bless my friends reading this right now. I am asking You to minister to their spirit at this very moment. Where there is pain, give them Your peace and mercy. Where there is self-doubting, release a renewed confidence in Your ability to work through them. Where there is tiredness, or exhaustion, I ask You to give them understanding, patience, and strength as they learn submission to Your leading. Where there is spiritual stagnation I ask You to renew them by revealing Your nearness, and by drawing them into greater intimacy with You. Where there is fear, reveal Your love, and release to them Your courage.

Where there is sin blocking them, reveal it and break its hold over my friends' life. Bless their finances, give them greater vision and raise up leaders, and friends to support, and encourage them. Give each of them discernment to recognize the power of You to help them in their life and healing.

Feb 19, 2003---

Today our doctors told us we could take a month off and go find some sun. They want to give the chemo and radiation a chance to work during that period of time. They said we should just go and don't think about it for a month. Our appointments are set for the cat scan, and as far as I know, there is nothing else we should do between now and then. We will continue our alternative procedures, and we will continue to ask for your wonderful prayers and support. After we take care of a few loose ends, we plan to load up the rig (that's our motor home), and head south. Thanks to all of you, and we'll keep you informed.

Feb 24, 2003---Dear Family and Friends,

Our plans have changed. We met with our doctor of natural medicine today, and found out that she has developed a treatment program for us that entails at least 2 treatments/week, between now and the end of March. She believes we can completely get rid of the tumor, between now and then. We've been working with her all along and we have a great deal of faith in her abilities. So we're going to stay home and keep fighting until April 2nd, when we have the cat scan. We're disappointed about postponing our trip, but we're convinced this is the best way to go. We'll just start our journey in April after Kathy is completely healed. Once again, thank you for your prayers and messages. We really appreciate them and we really still need them.

March 3, 2003----Dear Friends and Family,

Since we're staying here for treatments, we decided to move Kathy's catscan up to March 19th, with the doctor's evaluation set for March 25th. Kathy has been doing better, but on Saturday, doubts began creeping in and she started feeling quite anxious about the results of the cat scan. This, I'm told is common at this stage of the battle. We are concerned, because we believe we have to have total confidence that we're well, if we're going to win this battle. We decided to once again ask you all to keep us in your prayers, and especially pray for Kathy to overcome her fear and doubts, to regain her confidence in a complete cure. The night is sometimes darkest just before the dawn, and I believe that is the case now. But we need your continued help to see us through to victory. Kathy is strong and very brave, but sometimes it gets difficult when the battle gets long and tedious. Thank you again for all your support!

Mar 4, 2003---(here is a prayer sent from my mom's sister to her)

Dear God our Heavenly Father, please release Kathy from her fears and anxiety. Fill her with your spirit that brings comfort and peace. Your divine love surrounds her, and folds her and wraps her and she is relaxed and at peace, poised, balanced, serene and calm. The healing intelligence of her subconscious mind which created her body is now transforming every cell, nerve, tissue, muscle and bone of her being according to the perfect pattern of all organs lodged in her subconscious mind. Silently, quietly, all distorted thought patterns in her subconscious mind are removed and dissolved, and the vitality, wholeness, and beauty of the life principle are made manifest in every atom of her being. She is now open and receptive to the healing currents which are flowing through her like a river, restoring her to perfect health, harmony and peace. All distortions and ugly images are now washed away by the infinite ocean of love and peace flowing through her, and it is so. Thank you, Heavenly Father for your love.

Mar 5, 2003---(email from a relative who had also battled cancer)

Hi! I hope Kathy is feeling more positive about things, but remember always that when we aren't feeling the best, things have a way of not looking as good. I am a very positive person, but there were days when I just had to have someone understand how I really felt that minute. I needed someone to realize that I didn't always feel that way (like I was going to die, there was no way I could feel any better, etc.), but I wanted someone at that moment to just hold me and tell me it was ok to cry. I needed that freedom. I had been in the "Faith Movement" where we couldn't allow satan any room to work, and that was tough. I have worked with many people who have been in that, and the guilt was terrible. God knows what we feel inside anyway. He is bigger than any thoughts we may have. It is always important to think positively, that is a major part of the healing process. But God also gave us tears to use for our feelings and for feeling for those we love. I am praying that everything goes great when you have the cat scan. I hope all the treatments have done their thing and God has touched everything that has been done with His healing touch. It is a tough time for all of you. Waiting is so very hard, I am so glad that Kathy has such great supportive people holding her up at this time. That is so important. Knowing people cared was so important to me when I was sure I was going to die. I do pray that Kathy can remain positive about the cat scan and about her future. That is very important. More important is the love you have for each other and for God. That will get you through the toughest times even when things don't look so promising.

March 6, 2003---(email from another sister of my mom)

Hi...just wanted to pass on to you that I caught an interview on tv about a Dr. Weil, an M.D. who has written a number of books about natural healing. He is very impressive. His website is DrWeil.com. He addressed many health problems, and his knowledge of diseases, including cancer and its' treatment, both medical and natural, was amazing. Our thoughts and prayers are with you continually.

Mar 10, 2003---Dear Friends and Family,

The dark side has been rearing its ugly head lately, trying to frighten us into thinking we're not going to make it. I understand this can happen as we move closer and closer to success. We know what's happening, but it's still difficult to endure. We've initiated some new strategies this week, and I believe they will be helpful while we wait for the results of our treatments. The new experiences are as follows....

1. We met with Father Dale, a priest in town. He was recommended to us, and we had a very helpful talk with him about Kathy's condition. Both Kathy and I felt much better after our visit.

2. We went to a support group meeting and visited with three wonderful ladies who have cancer. I was so impressed with their courage and their loving ways of inspiring us to live with hope and optimism.

3. We hired a cook who comes to our house and prepares healthful, organic, vegetarian meals for us. I've never been much of a cook.

4. Our daughter taped a program from The Lakewood Church in Houston that dealt with the exact problem we are currently facing. The pastor is Joel Osteen and he discussed ways to remain faithful and stay positive in the face of any adversity. Our nephew took us

to the Lakewood church when we were in Houston, so we got to hear him in person. He is really inspiring and presents a useful message in every sermon.

Kathy is holding her own as far as weight is concerned, but she's not gaining as rapidly as I would like. She is eating more and more, and I'm sure it will start to show soon. We are still visiting our natural doctor once or twice/week, and Kathy also visited two massage therapists this week. Kathy continues to be strong and very brave during this ordeal. She says she can hardly wait until it's all over and she's well again. We really enjoy hearing from you all, and thanks for being there for us.

Mar 21, 2003---Dear Friends and Relatives,

We could feel your prayers and good wishes this morning, and our prayers were answered! Kathy's tumor looks like it was hit with a bunker-busting bomb. The doctors said that they are very pleased with what they see, but, they have a little disagreement about what to do next. The left lung has some residual necrosis, which is dead tumor cells. There is the possibility that there may be some cancer left in that residue, and that's where the doctors disagree. One doctor wants to do a bronchoscopy, and the other doctor thinks we should wait two months, and then do a pet scan, because the radiation is still working. They are conferring and will let us know what they recommend. We will continue with all our holistic treatments until we are absolutely certain the cancer is eradicated. Dr. Wright, our natural medicine doctor, said her treatments would turn the tumor to mush. It looks like that is what happened to it. Thank you all, and keep us in your thoughts and prayers...it really works!!!

Mar 24, 2003--- Dear Friends and Family,

Kathy will be having a bronchoscopy on Mar 28th. The doctors want to find out if any of the debris in Kathy's left lung contains live cancer cells. If it does, they'll want to administer more chemo. They don't think that's the case, but we're going to check, just to be sure. We won't know anything until the following week, and we'll let you know what we find out. Kathy is feeling better every day, and our only task now is to help her gain some of the weight back. She's been through the mill, and it takes a while to get the body and mind back to normalcy. We're continuing with our holistic treatments, as we believe it's the main reason for our success (after prayer, of course). We are going to see Dr. Wright, our doctor of natural medicine tomorrow for more treatments and consultation. Although we're happy with our apparent victory, we are being cautious. We plan to follow through on all our procedures until we are absolutely certain the cancer is totally gone. These treatments include prayer, and we hope you'll all continue to remember us in your prayers. Finally, we want to thank you all once again for your wonderful support during those dark days of January and February in what was the roughest winter of our lives. Your kind thoughts, prayers and messages were extremely helpful.

March 28, 2003---Dear Friends and Relatives,

Kathy's bronchoscopy went well today. The doctor looked in her left lung and said it looks like dead cells and no cancer. He took several biopsies and will call us next week with the results. The only way to know for sure is by doing the biopsies. We need your help to get Kathy to eat more so she can increase her weight. Her weight is down to 100 pounds, and she is having trouble believing the good news. We are really concerned. We think we beat the cancer, but now we're dealing with this problem. Your prayers and ideas are always welcome. More later, have a nice weekend.

April 1, 2003---Dear Friends and Family,

Thank you all for efforts to rid Kathy of cancer. The doctor called and told us he saw NO SIGN of cancer in Kathy's left lung. It's the best news we could possibly get! He said we should continue to watch it carefully, because cancer has a way of coming back. We plan to continue our treatments, and most importantly, our prayers. God gave us a second chance, and we plan to make the most of it. Our entire family will be eternally grateful to all of you for your wonderful support. Our love and prayers to you...

April 1, 2003---(email from my mom's sister)

We are absolutely thrilled that you are cancer free, and can now go on looking forward to the future without this cloud. We will keep you in our thoughts and prayers always, Thank God for this blessing!

April 1, 2003---(email from another of my mom's sisters)

It's a miracle from God! I can't tell you how unbelievably happy I am. What you went through was the toughest, most unbearable experience; but you prevailed!! We'll all be eternally grateful for your strength and God's blessing.

April 1, 2003 (email from a family friend)

What great news! You are truly blessed. I can hardly wait to share the news with my prayer group today...we love to hear those answers to prayers. Praise God from whom all blessings flow!

April 1, 2003---(email from my mom's sister)

It's such great news!! And we are so grateful for our answered prayers...we share in your joy and give thanks to our Heavenly Father. SLEEP WELL...............

In conclusion, my mom was cured of cancer thanks to the grace of God, and to a lesser extent, natural and traditional methods. We are forever thankful to all the friends, relatives, doctors (including everyone at the hospital who aided mom in many ways), and Dr. Wright for her natural methods of curing my mom as well. We thank my dad's chiropractor also for suggesting Dr. Wright to us. Without Dr. Wright, my mom's comfort would have been greatly reduced during this ordeal. I am very proud of my mom for being such a strong person and fighting through the nightmare of cancer. My dad was an incredible help to my mom through this, and I am very grateful to him as well.

My whole family helped in every way they could, and we all are so happy to have my mom back in good health these 10 years since the cancer was destroyed. Another thing we did that helped a lot when she was going through her treatment and recovery and even to this day is we went to a religious goods store and bought figurines of saints, guardian angels, little cards with biblical sayings on them, and a big gold plaque that we hung on the wall that says "BE STILL AND KNOW THAT I AM". All of these items were and are constant reminders of God and His love and caring for us. They were very comforting during mom's most difficult days. We still have them out to this day, and feel comforted by them now too, in our daily lives. I hope this book has helped give you hope and strength in your journey and that it will ultimately help you get cured of cancer forever. Many good wishes and blessings to you........